EARS THAT DON'T WORK RIGHT

STORIES FROM THE HEART

WHAT IT'S LIKE TO LIVE IN A WORLD WHERE YOU CAN'T DEPEND ON THE WORDS YOU HEAR & HOW HEARING AIDS CHANGED EVERYTHING

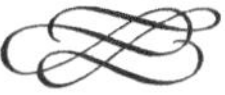

DR. DEVON HUNING, AU.D.

FOREWORD

I spent 30+ years of my life as an audiologist, working with people of all ages, from many cultures, financial backgrounds and educations. They all shared one thing in common…hearing loss had a huge negative impact on their lives. Socially, emotionally, economically, educationally. It crept into all corners. And sadly, at one time or another, they all also experienced the same reactions from their friends, family, spouses, parents, co-workers, clerks. Those of impatience - "oh,, never mind!", criticism - "you're not listening!", judgment - "what are you, deaf??!"

For dare I say all other impairments or handicaps, others show at least a modicum of compassion, sympathy or patience. But not hearing loss.

After so many years, I think I finally figured out that it is because hearing loss is invisible, and we humans need to be able to see, feel or touch something to believe it's really true. Well, I'm sorry, but you'll just have to wear some earplugs for a day to *feel* a tiny bit of what it's like not to hear and that's as close as you'll get. Otherwise, you'll have to take the stories in this book as notice of what it's really like to live in a world where most of what you hear is a struggle to understand. Where everyone sounds like they have a mouthful of marbles, and where struggling to understand is sometimes just too hard.

This book is dedicated to my patients who, over the years, gave me back more than they will ever know. Moments when a little girl began to sing the first time she heard her own voice, or when a simple device recommended to an RVing couple "saved our marriage", or when a woman hugged me after saying "You've given me my life back," after fitting her with hearing aids. There's nothing harder than telling parents their child has hearing loss, and nothing more gratifying than supporting them through their journey of acceptance. The newborns, the toddlers, the teens, the young and old men and women,, thank you. There are so many, but I hope sharing these few stories helps the hearing world understand your struggles, the pitfalls of hearing loss and discover the patience and compassion that lies within us all.

DS

Being hearing-impaired from my point of view:

- Quality of life - 2 out of 5.
- People have no patience with you when you have to ask them to repeat.
- Trying to work with the public is very difficult. Miss hearing their words.
- Unable to even watch the news, a movie, etc. in comfort as voices all muffled.
- As hearing became its worst, just decided to opt out of a lot of events, as it became too frustrating trying to cope. Everyday things like shopping and family gatherings became very difficult as I couldn't understand voices when in crowds.
- I found over time I had no focus and was becoming depressed and upset with the inability to communicate properly.

Kept putting off seeking hearing aids mostly due to the expense. Maybe now that I have hearing aids, life will get back on track. Thank you.

RB

Got my new hearing aids. Wow! Really opened my ears to all the sounds I forgot were even there. Hearing my own footsteps, birds singing, trees creaking in the wind…just to name a few. So much thanks!

SO

I struggle to understand speech even in quiet without my hearing aids. I can't hear the "ding" of the microwave, the phone ringing, rain, wind, birdsongs, the higher registers of a church organ, the drip of the kitchen faucet, crickets and piccolos, when I'm not wearing my hearing aids. My world is devoid of many environmental sounds and is very quiet without my hearing aids. I only hear the "swishing sound" of whispered voices. If you get my attention and face me while speaking to me, I will better be able to understand what you're saying to me by "speech reaching". Are hearing aids perfect? No, they're not. Hearing aids don't "correct" our hearing the same way glasses "correct" our vision. People with hearing loss have to make a conscious effort to hear media they are interested in. Listening fatigue is real. People who have not experienced hearing loss don't understand that increased volume doesn't help me to hear any better. So please don't tell me to turn up my hearing aids or insist I see my audiologist for an adjustment.

Deafness is a much worse misfortune. For it means the loss of the most viral stimulus-the sound of the voice that brings language, sets thoughts astir, and keeps us in the intellectual company of man.

— HELEN KELLER

TH

A freak accident, the tree branch punctured my ear drum and ear canal that day. The ensuing infection and complications from this wound left me with a severe hearing loss, tinnitus and a different life. Not at all what I'd expected from helping at Grandpa's farm that day! .... "Mrs. H, there's nothing more we can do for Tommy.......he'll have to get a hearing aid."

For a time, my balance was affected, so I walked kind of funny. I had some headaches, and an awful "buzzing" sound. When spoken to on the right side, unless it was loud, I could just hear "mush". Normally congenial and chatty, I got very tired of having folks repeat words, phrases and sentences. And folks got tired of helping. My wide circle of friends got smaller, I was not included and became very sad about it. Instead of dreading a hearing aid, I was actually looking forward to it! Hoping it would return things to normal, clearing up sounds, particularly on which side they were coming from. Maybe having more friends again?

In those days [1960's], hearing aids were fitted by specialty offices [NOT audiologists!]. ...... "Mrs. H. like Dr. said, Tommy has suffered a serious injury to his right ear...... how bad said Grandma........Mrs. H. Tommy has the hearing like a 70 year old man...." Good news is that we have a hearing aid that will help.

In November of 1967 I was fitted with my first hearing aid. I was so excited, scared, apprehensive and likely awkward......my hopes were to put it on and things would clear up. I wished for a cure.

Oh, my, I could hear sound again! The buzzing stopped! The initial dislike of the device and fear I had about looking strange and different went away! I am sure he showed the operation of the hearing aid, but I forgot as I marveled at how great it was to hear...

My first big public outing was to go to church with mom on a Sunday. I can so remember the church folk coming up to my mother to express their sadness with words like, "Oh, moms name, I'm so sorry for Tommy...." "I didn't know it was THAT BAD". Like I'd gotten some terrible illness... Back then, hearing loss needing amplification was almost shameful.......what I thought was a relief, could actually become a curse. It was a sure sign of a defect, age, illness or physical weakness. Jokes were made, teasing and worse. Folks did not know how to speak to me, very loud? SLOWWW and simple? Or worse, not at all......."Oh never mind"......GRRR.

It's been that way for 56 years. In today's polite society, no one would ever mock or make fun of a blind person or a disability. Why oh why do we allow and encourage jokes, cartoons making fun of hearing loss?

Kindness is the language which the deaf can hear and the blind can see.

— *MARK TWAIN*

ES

Hearing problem - something I would not wish on anyone. You may be talking to someone about something and you are not getting half of what he or she is telling you, very embarrassing. I've been there.

I am a musician and I play with a church group. I play guitar and button accordion. Many times I am too loud or I am not loud enough. I can't tell because I am not hearing how loud my music is. Not good.

I also find that your balance is not like it should be and it may stop you from doing things that you always did. Those are some of the problems I find in having a hearing problem. Thank God for hearing aids!

EW

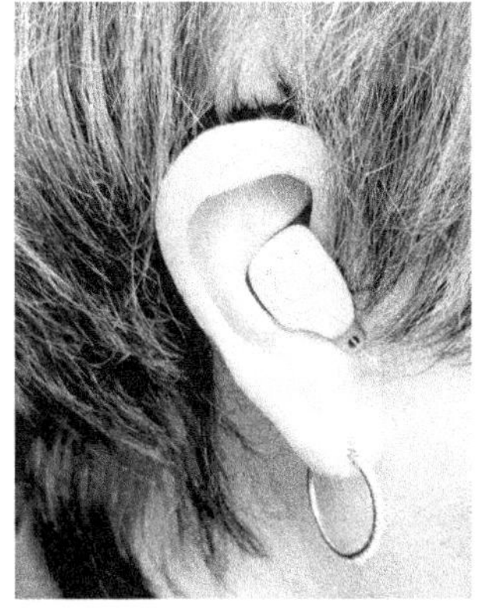

In my 60's I realized I was having difficulty hearing. I felt very frustrated and isolated. There were many things I could not participate in, including lively conversations. We sometimes don't realize how many activities we are exempt from when we have a hearing loss.

After receiving my hearing aids, I found so many differences. I could now participate in many activities and be involved. My hearing is not restored to the original but I am thankful and blessed every day because I hear as well as I do.

PR

It was approximately 2 years ago that my husband, family members and of course, myself noticed something had changed. I was, however, going through a denial period and trying to convince myself that it was other issues, such as blocked passages, wax, etc.

As time went on, it became very obvious that there was a problem - hearing loss. I became very depressed. I booked an appointment for a hearing test. During the examination, my thoughts led me to believe it was going to be ok! …it wasn't!

I was withdrawn and as I said, depressed. My first experience with hearing aids was a total disaster! However, through a friend, God led me to the most precious professional lady that worked with me through the ups and downs. I am pleased with my new aids. Yes, it's a big adjustment to one's life - but there's help!

Sweet is every sound, sweeter the voice, but every sound is sweet.

— *ALFRED LLOYD TENNYSON*

DH

I am 39 years old. I have been suffering from hearing loss since I was a little girl. In total, I've had approximately 13 surgeries on my ears. When I was 16, I did try to go to hearing aids; however, they caused more trouble than anything as they blocked off air flow through my ear which caused moisture to accumulate causing me to continue getting multiple ear infections.

In 2020, I had my last surgery. I decided that was it, no more. I was used to living with hearing loss and as long as it remained the same, I should be good, living a "normal" life. Unfortunately, then COVID struck and everyone began wearing masks. I realized then how much I depended on lip reading. I decided then that I had no other option than to try hearing aids once again.

Since going forward with hearing aids, my life has increasingly improved. I was amazed to realize how little I could actually hear. Little things like rain falling, a knock on the door, even the dishwasher running. I was in awe with how noisy the world actually was!

I can tell now how frustrating it was when I would continuously ask "What?" to those around me. Or seeing my little boy taking a frustrated breath of air when I couldn't hear what he was saying. And those saying "Never mind." because they have repeated what they said 3 times already.

You start feeling like a burden for them to be having to continuously repeat themselves, like you're annoying people.

When I wear my hearing aids, I actually feel proud to be a part of the conversation. If you ask my husband, he will boast about how happy he is when I wear them. He immediately knows the minute he talks to me if I'm not wearing them. He stops the conversation and tells me to go put them in.

My aids are becoming one of the most important technologies in my life. I don't think I could ever go back to life without them.

PI

Yesterday, I forgot my hearing aids. I had to go to the dentist and went for coffee. A man was sitting next to me and I couldn't understand a word! It's frustrating when you can't hear someone! With my hearing aids on, I'm very comfortable.

But what a humiliation for me when someone standing next to me heard a flute in the distance and I heard nothing, or someone standing next to me heard a shepherd singing and again I heard nothing. Such incidents drove me almost to despair - a little more of that and I would have ended my life. It was only my art that held me back.

— *LUDWIG VAN BEETHOVEN*

FO

I didn't realize I had any problem hearing until I found I could not hear the TV as well and at my children's homes the TV was too low for me. Since getting my hearing aids, it's been amazing! I can hear and the sound is great.

SK

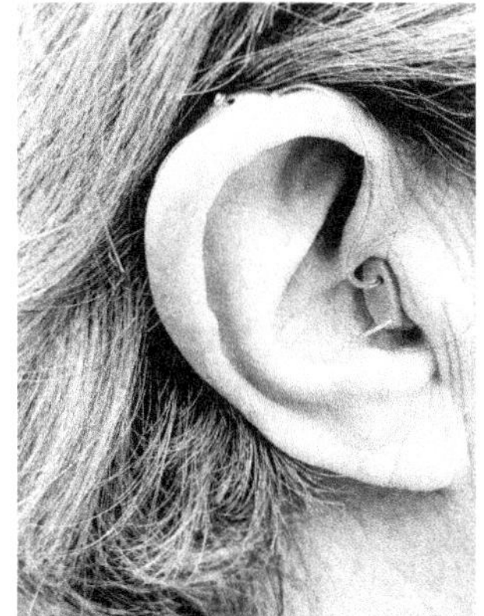

I am so happy to be able to hear better without hearing muffled words. I know I would and should have had the aids much sooner. Thank you for your patience with me!

DF

Without my hearing aids, I am totally lost. It's not good when you are home alone and someone knocks on your door and you don't hear them and they do frighten you. I can hear a lot better with two hearing aids than just one. It seems with one, you are just getting bits and pieces of the conversation. Thank you so much!

YW

Loss of hearing? No, not me! I am hearing fine as I thought. Nope…I was not hearing fine at all. My biggest difference that hearing aids made for me was at my work place. The girls at the office used to repeat things to me all the time. They thought I wasn't hearing but no one would say anything to me about it.They would ask me "You got that, didn't you?" If I didn't, they would repeat it. I guess I trained myself in lip reading and didn't even notice it. The big problem came when we had to wear masks all the time. I then realized that the mask was making me nearly deaf - I thought I was going deaf all the time!

I can honestly say that I love wearing my hearing aids! I don't have to ask the second time…can you repeat that please? I'm more engaged in conversations than ever before in places like conferences, church, shopping or wherever there is a group of people. It could get really funny some days…no more funny remarks or incidents now!

PP

It's frustrating. You just can't understand things when you can't hear. You're in a world where you're not present. You can only communicate using your hands. You feel lost. With hearing aids, it's a different world. You can hear in ways that make a big difference.

The first time I got my hearing aids, when I got in the car, I heard the turn signal for the first time. The toilet flushing, more environmental sounds were awesome.

It was a big step getting hearing aids. Before, I could hear things but not understand. With my implant, even only on one side, I'm hearing amazing sounds in the environment I've never heard. It's unreal! My implant and my hearing aid together, it's sooooo good!

RW

For many years, I had been contending with a hearing problem, finding it very uncomfortable and hard to hear as I should. I would have to turn the TV up really high to get what was being said. I found it really hard to hear on the telephone. For me, the routine was continually asking people to repeat what they said.

My grandchildren would get much amusement from the fact that they would ask me questions and I would give them extremely unrelated answers because I could not hear them properly. Whereas, they being grandchildren, would laugh, other people would just smile…

Hearing loss can affect your whole well being. It can put a damper on an individual's self esteem. I am sure that the bird's melody and singing didn't sound as beautiful to me as it does now.

My hearing problem wasn't inherited from my mother for sure, who passed away in her 101st year, and right up to that point, she had excellent hearing!

She could hear and understand what everybody said, could hear the slightest pin when it dropped to the floor and could hear the faintest whisper.

Since I got hearing aids, I can now hear people talking more clearly, can hear the kettle boiling, hear the clock ticking, can hear my footsteps (which was probably one of the most noticeable). People don't have to shout any more for me to hear them. Also, I, myself, don't talk as loud. Like the slogan "Things go better with coke.", all in all... Things... life in general, goes better with hearing aids!

Hearing is a form of touch. You feel it through your body, and sometimes it almost hits your face.

— *EVELYN GLENNIE*

GR

I feel very blessed to have received hearing aids. They have made a remarkable difference in my life! I now hear sounds very crisp and clean.

CAH

For years, I missed out on a lot of people talking to me and not hearing what they were saying. I didn't know if I should answer "yes" or "no" to what they were saying. Now, it's delightful just to hear things I would normally miss. My hearing aids are the best things I ever purchased. I couldn't believe how beautiful the wind could sound until I had my hearing aids…

CM

Hearing is much more precise [with hearing aids], especially words that sound alike. Sounds of music - fantastic! Clear and overall a much greater improvement than not having them!

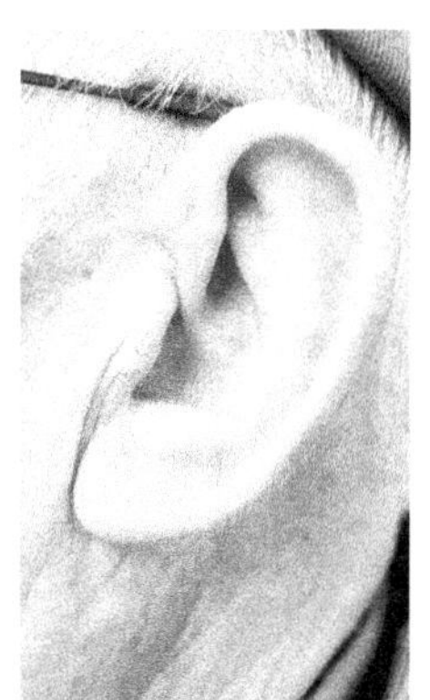

BM

I realize the small sounds I've not been hearing. With my hearing aids, they have made such a difference with my tinnitus. When I remove them at night, I realize just how loud it is.

~

AP

Hearing aids changed my life. I didn't realize how noisy the world was until I had them. And also how quiet it could be when the ringing stopped. Makes life so much better!

The thing about hearing loss is that no one can see it. Most people are so impatient, they just assume that the person with hearing loss is being rude or slow-witted.

— *MARION ROSS*

JM

It was embarrassing when someone would be talking to me on my left side, and I couldn't even hear them. I didn't realize they were talking to me. It has had a profound effect, being able to hear on both sides again! It has greatly enhanced my well-being and confidence, especially in social settings.

Not having to have the television up on a high volume is certainly better for my husband. He always said the TV was so high and I didn't even know…

I am so grateful that my hearing has vastly improved. I love my hearing aids!!!

K

Received my new hearing aids about a year ago. Life changing… I didn't realize what I was missing. They are so comfortable that you actually forget you have them on. I was talking to a friend of mine who wanted and needed aids, but was too embarrassed. I told him it is the best investment he could make!

To go outside and listen to the wind blow and hear the rain is awesome. When I walked my dog before hearing aids, I was always looking behind me to see if a car was coming. But now, I hear the car before it gets up to us.

Talking to people in a crowd is different. You don't have to smile and nod your head *as if* you understand because you actually do!

MK

I had forgotten the name of a friend's son after someone asked me. Outside in my garden, I called out to my daughter because I knew she knew his name. She turned around and I heard her say "Dot!".

"Dot", I said. That's not his name. I called out again..." What's his name?"

"Dot! Dot!" she yelled. Finally, she came right up to my face and said "Scot! S-C-O-T! Put on your hearing aids mom!"

KJ

Since getting my hearing aids, my life has gotten so much better. I can now be in a crowd and feel included in the conversations. When at work, I don't have to ask clients to repeat what they have said and my fellow employees don't have to yell or repeat what they have said a million times. Hearing aids have improved my life 100%!

Listening is a magnetic and strange thing, a creative force.

— *KARL A. MENNINGER*

MM

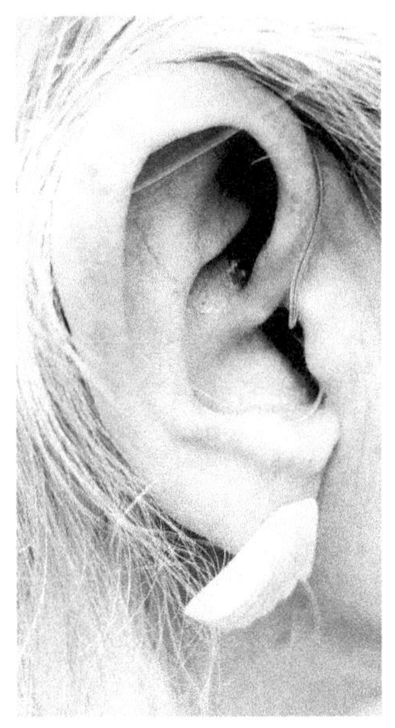

When I was watching a movie, I could hear one character quite plainly. When the next one would speak, it was all gibberish, couldn't understand a word! And I couldn't understand *why* I could understand one person but not the other. When listening to the radio, a song would come on with loud music and I would say "They're just bawlin', just sayin' words," because I couldn't understand a word!

I remember once when my son and his wife came home and they were sitting by me, talkin' away. I couldn't understand a word and that's what I told them. I thought to myself...how can they hear each other and I don't understand? It was all very frustrating. I thought "What's wrong with me? How come I don't understand?"

A lot of people would speak to me and I would say "What?" all the time. They'd hardly be finished with what they were saying before I'd be saying "What?" At some point I caught on that if I waited a few seconds I would get what they said. But I didn't get it right from the beginning.

All that changed when I got hearing aids. I could finally hear the characters in a movie. The next time my son and his wife came over, I could follow the conversation. Now, I don't say "What???" so often! And it's such a relief, not to have to say "What did you say?" all the time!

MW

I first noticed my hearing loss when not being able to completely understand TV and radio conversations without turning up the volume. Also, I was having to continually ask people to repeat what they had said. Telephone conversations were getting worse as well, to the point that I would not answer the phone if the call display showed certain people who were not a crisp, clear speaker. I blamed their mumbling…

My bosses's wife was hearing-impaired and she suggested a hearing test. Thankfully, I followed her advice.

I can't believe the difference [now that I have hearing aids]. I'm more confident on the phone and I actually can hear the birds chirp. Awesome! Before, people had no trouble sneaking up behind me to scare me, jokingly, but they rarely succeed now! My suggestion to anyone experiencing anything like I did - get the test!

Several times a day, stop and just listen.

— *JAN CHOZEN BAYS*

EK

It was very difficult for me, not hearing, before I got my hearing aids. I would constantly be asking people what they were saying. I couldn't join in a conversation if we had company over. It was very frustrating.

Since getting them, I can hear and join in the conversation. I haven't had to say "What are you saying?" for a while. Really glad I have them!

BM

I didn't realize that I couldn't hear everyone, but my children told me over and over that I should get my hearing checked. I ignored them for a year or more but finally gave in just to prove them wrong!

Boy was I surprised. My hearing aids opened a new way of life for me. I was more confident in group discussions. I could hear sounds I never realized were around me.

Don't hesitate. It doesn't mean getting old - it means keeping in contact with everyone.

DE

Before, when I couldn't hear, I felt left out in a lot of things because I couldn't hear conversations. It got to the point that I stopped going out.

Since getting my hearing aids, it's amazing. I never knew how much I had been missing - birds chirping, rain on the roof, kids playing. It was like a whole new world - and I'm still being amazed! Now I can hear my 19-month-old granddaughter talking to me. For that, I am very, very grateful.

CB

I have heard things that I haven't heard in a long time. Didn't really know I *couldn't* hear them until I got my hearing aids…Best move I ever made!

> *At some point we have to stop and say "There's Marlee." Not, "There's the deaf actress."*
>
> — *MARLEE MATLIN*

WM

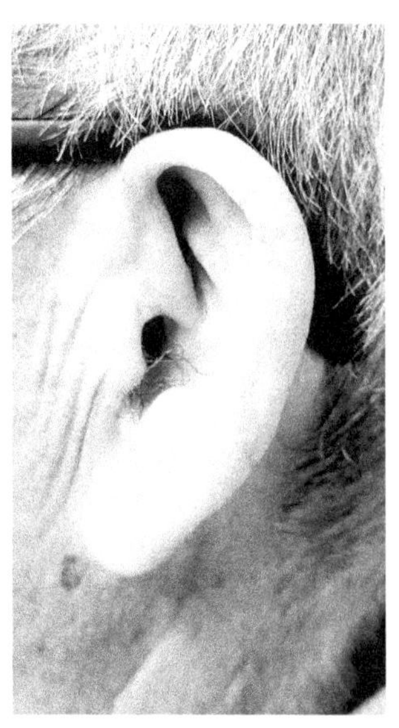

I guess it was a gradual process of the loss of my hearing and I just didn't realize the situation. I'm hearing things now that I thought would be no more.

I can hear my footsteps, like the crunching of snow or the sand or gravel when I walk. Many other sounds have come to life. I can understand conversations much better, especially with the grandchildren. I now know how many "Can you do this…?" or "Can you do that…?" directions I get from my better half!

DW

Prior to aids, many times conversations would not be received in my head. My answers were incorrect and I would back away from conversations with people. During a party, I did not get half of a conversation, thus I would miss the meaning.

The first day I used the aids and I walked out of this building, the sound of sand under my shoes amazed me!

Leaves near our house sounded perfect, along with the sound of birds - music to my ears!

AL

Hearing aids! Did I really need them? I struggled with the idea for quite some time until finally I decided to pursue the idea and see an audiologist. I soon realized that my hearing loss was certainly evident. However, I was gradually losing hearing and it was causing multiple problems.

After 12 months of wearing hearing aids, my whole life changed. Now, I am able to have conversations with family, friends, etc. This was quite amazing indeed!

I am now aware that the whole component of the hearing concept has changed so much of my daily life. Yes, I hear sounds that were almost non-existent. Hearing aids have changed so many things that make everything seem so natural. If you ever need hearing aids, go for them! You will see and hear life in a new dimension.

I have the right to listen and hear.

— *ANONYMOUS*

GK

Without my hearing aids, I am almost completely adrift. It is very frightening when they are out. Everything is so good when I put them in. It would be a different world without them. I can almost feel what people without their hearing feel like…

~

BN

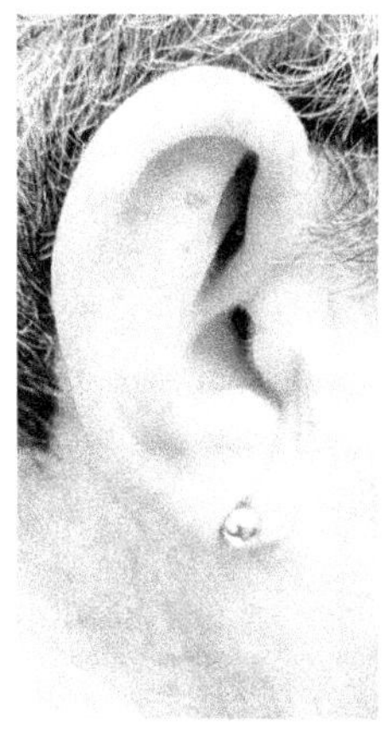

Frustration! Constantly asking people to repeat. Not hearing announcements. Hearing aids have kept me from being locked out of things. Are they perfect? By no means. But they help. All people working with the general public need to be taught how to be clear. Most turn and walk away when speaking, leaving you with no clue as to what to do.

~

ME

Now that I have hearing loss, I can understand why my dad became more subdued, quiet and withdrawn from social settings.

When you constantly ask to repeat, you are embarrassed and stop communicating. You tend to prefer reading activities and less watching TV. A quieter life, less distractions and noise, and clarity of speech!

VK

It is difficult to live with someone with hearing loss. Everything has to be repeated and it gets frustrating. Also, there is a fear that if the other person gets sick and the hearing aids are not in, then the person won't be able to hear. It is embarrassing for the person with the hearing loss when everything has to be repeated.

An elderly man was having hearing problems and went to see a specialist. The doctor fitted him with some hearing aids that brought his hearing back to full strength.

After a few weeks the man came back to make sure the new equipment was working properly, which it was.

The hearing specialist said, "It all seems perfect. Your family should be delighted you can hear everything now."

"Oh no," the man responded. "I haven't told any of them. I just sit quietly, listening carefully. I've changed my will four times."

SD

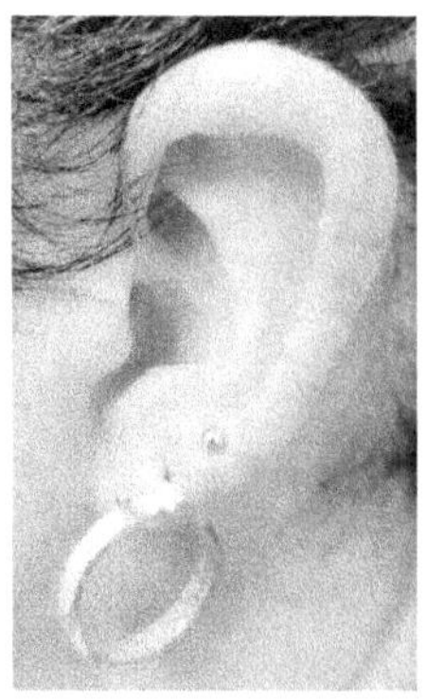

I was in my early 20's when I discovered I had hearing loss. It was quite scary at the time and I couldn't imagine myself wearing hearing aids. I went on for years, refusing to use hearing aids but struggling to hear and understand conversations around me. I would ask people to repeat themself a LOT! I found myself relying heavily on lipreading and needing to see the person's face and lips to hear. It came to the point where I would avoid certain situations related to my hearing.

Finally, my audiologist put it to me like this... *"Without hearing aids, your brain will begin to forget sounds and words, conversations will become much more difficult."* I think that I felt getting hearing aids would be an admission of my disability. But with more time, he finally convinced me that hearing aids were a necessity for my hearing health as well as my quality of life.

Hearing aids have changed my life for the better. They did take some getting used to and there are days I despise them, but without them, I would be lost. When you can't hear or have to ask someone to repeat, in a way you feel stupid. Hearing aids can give you the confidence you need to socialize and live your life!

EH

I notice that quite often, unfortunately, those who hear well are quite impatient with their loved ones who do not hear well. They get annoyed if they have to repeat themselves or if the hearing-impaired person just doesn't get what's being said. People don't show the same annoyance to the visually impaired. They are treated so differently!

I also notice when I am at concerts, etc., I see people laughing at jokes, etc., so I laugh along with them - but I didn't hear the joke…I do not like always whispering "What was that???"

But, since my hearing aids, I hear so much better!

Mr. Smith suspects his wife is hard of hearing. He decides to test this. As his wife is chopping vegetables in the kitchen, he stands 10 feet behind her and says softly, "Honey, what's for dinner?" There is no response, so he moves a step closer and asks more loudly, "Honey, what's for dinner?" She keeps chopping vegetables, so he steps even closer, raises his voice and says, "Honey, what's for dinner?" Hearing nothing, he starts to step even closer when she turns around and says, "Dear, I said 'chicken and salad' three times!"

BW

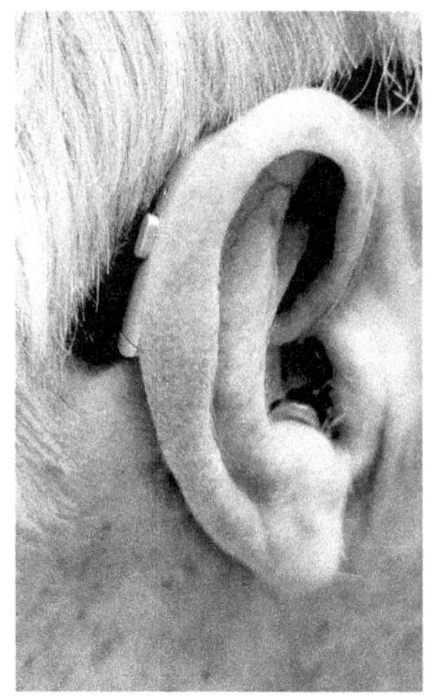

Hearing to me is so very important in my life. Sitting at the table and not being able to join in a conversation is so depressing. You feel left out because you want to be a part of that conversation.

With hearing aids, they make you feel a part of the group and so happy to join in on the conversation. They can be a nuisance at times in having to change batteries and clean them, but having them outweighs all this by a lot!

Enjoy people, enjoy life, enjoy a wonderful conversation, hear the beautiful sounds of life. If you need them, get them!

Difficulty hearing with or without hearing aids is no joke. Untreated hearing loss can lead to earlier onset of cognitive decline, balance issues resulting in more falls, difficulties telling where sounds are coming from causing safety issues, and so much more.

If you or someone you know suspects hearing loss, please see an audiologist in your area for a complete audiological assessment.

I hope you enjoyed these stories. They came from the heart of the people that wrote them and what their lives are like not being able to hear. And best of all, how much better their quality of life became once they got hearing aids.

It would mean a lot to me if you would take just a few moments to go back to Amazon and leave an honest review of this book. Thank you, and all the best wherever your journey takes you!

Scan the QR code below to leave a review on Amazon.

A few communication tips for the hearing and the hard-of-hearing.

For the hearing:

- Face the person you're talking to - **room-to-room conversations don't work!**
- When possible, minimize the background noise. What might be music to you is 'noise' to the hard-of-hearing.
- If repetition is requested, don't be a parrot. Try to rephrase what you've said.
- Try speaking in short phrases with barely perceptible pauses. Google "clear speech" and you'll get an idea of what it is and how to do it.
- When out to eat, don't cover your mouth so you can talk with your mouth full. Just don't talk with your mouth full.
- Avoid the middle of the room like it was the black hole of death. As far as communication goes, that's what it is! Try to sit on the perimeter, and even in a corner or a booth if available.
- The same is true for any crowded room. If you're having a conversation with a hard-of-hearing person, steer them to the side of the room.

For the hard-of-hearing:

- Yes, for best results, you still have to face each other even with your aids on!
- If you need to ask for repetition, try this. Someone asks you *"Do you want to go to dinner on Friday?"* but

you didn't get it. Instead of saying "*What did you say?*", respond with "*I got something about dinner. What was the rest of it?*" That way, the other person knows how better to help you.

- If you think or know you do have hearing loss, don't put off getting help any longer.
- Some of the same tips for people with normal hearing will help you, too!
- Don't be afraid to tell people you have trouble hearing and then tell them how they can help - speak a little more slowly, oh, please don't yell, can you repeat that with different words, etc.
- If your hearing is better in one ear than the other, arrange communication settings so that side is favored.

www.ingramcontent.com/pod-product-compliance
Lightning Source LLC
Chambersburg PA
CBHW071251150726
48001CB00018B/1094

* 9 7 9 8 3 4 9 3 7 3 2 3 7 *